LIVING WITH A COLECTOMY: A GUIDE FOR FAMILIES, 2ND EDITION

Roberta Schneider

ISBN: 9798858437253
Printed in the United States of America

INTRODUCTION

I never expected shoulder pain to lead us down this journey.

It started with a phone call from a chiropractor, canceling my husband's appointment, sending him to his primary care physician and telling him that something on his X-ray was very, very wrong.

This started weeks of bouncing among specialists trying to find out a solution to fix an extremely serious health situation. My husband's lung had collapsed, his colon had grown to roughly 5 times the normal size and encroached on the lung space, moving over his heart. Multiple surgeries were going to be needed to help return him to normal. By the time of the first surgery, the colon was causing serious issues with his ability to breathe, so much that walking up the stairs or tying shoes were difficult. We recognized quickly that we were a medical anomaly but the steps needed to resolve this to help return his life to normal were not unique.

As we began to research what would happen at each stage, we were surprised by the lack of educational resources and support for patients after each surgery.

We could easily learn what would happen from a technical standpoint during the colectomy, also known as colon resection surgery, and that supposedly my husband could start returning to normal activity in a few weeks. But gaps existed when it came to what to truly expect in that recovery phase. We've learned firsthand the impacts a colon resection surgery can have on a person's diet, sleep, activity, work and relationships.

Your health journey may be different than ours. Your journey with colon surgery may be prompted by irritable bowel disease. Or colon cancer. Or diverticulitis. Or Chron's disease. But the common denominator is the reality of living with a colectomy.

For the 600,000 people who have this type of colon surgery each year, a colectomy can be life-changing, not just for you but for your loved ones as well. Nationally, one in five adults is assisting someone as an unpaid caregiver. This means additional financial stress, dietary and lifestyle changes, as well as helping someone through a surgery recovery process. That doesn't include the impacts on every child and adult living in your household.

This guide, based on research from national and international experts on colon and gastrointestinal issues, as well as our family's experiences after colon resection surgery, is designed to help you navigate the changes as a family. This process may feel like the loneliest journey, but you are not alone.

THE BASICS OF A COLECTOMY

A colectomy, or colon resection surgery, is when part or all of your colon is removed from your digestive system. The remaining parts of your colon are reconnected so your body can continue to have bowel movements to get rid of wastes.

Your colorectal surgeon or general surgeon might recommend you need a colectomy for a number of reasons such as:

- A birth defect in the colon
- Blockage in the colon
- Chron's disease
- Colon cancer
- Colon stricture (a colon that is narrowed)
- Colon that is twisted
- Diverticulitis
- Hirschrung's disease
- Inflammatory bowel disease
- Polyps in colon
- Ulcerative colitis

Depending on your medical condition, all or part of your

colon may be removed in the colon resection surgery. The surgery may be done in an "open" manner with a long incision, or "minimally invasive," which involves several small incisions in your abdomen and typically has a shorter recovery time.

Your colon, also known as the large intestine, has one job: moving the food waste from the small intestine. This long, muscular tube squeezes the water from the waste and pushes the remaining waste to the rectum so you can have a bowel movement.

But what happens when part of your colon is removed?

Your body still has to get rid of the solid waste, and that needs to find a way out somehow. To allow solid waste to be removed from your body, your surgeon will do one of these options during a colectomy:

- Rejoin the remaining portions of your colon, called an anastomosis. This keeps your waste going through your body.
- Connect your intestine to an opening in your abdomen, called a stoma. This lets your waste leave your body through an attached colostomy bag, which can be used temporarily or permanently.
- Removing both the colon and rectum and connecting your small intestine to your anus in a total colectomy.

Surgeries are never without risk. Colectomies are no different. Complications of a colectomy include:

- Bleeding
- Blood clots in the legs or lungs
- Hernia
- Ileus, or the inability for your intestines to contract

- Infection
- Injury to organs near your colon, such as the bladder and small intestines
- Leakage
- Tears in the sutures that reconnect the remaining parts of your digestive system

While doctors say having a colectomy can have a relatively short recovery period of a few weeks, the reality is colon resection can be a life-altering surgery.

Tips For Talking With Your Colorectal Surgeon

Being told you need to have colon resection surgery - or any surgery, for that matter - can make you feel concerned. It's natural to have many questions about what to expect before, during and after your colon surgery.

Not everyone feels comfortable talking with a surgeon or other healthcare providers. The following tips can help you get ready to talk with your doctor. By planning ahead you can feel more comfortable with your pre-surgery or post-surgery visit.

- Before each appointment, write down your main concerns and a list of questions. These may be about the procedure, side effects, mental health, or short-term disability or FMLA papers. Ask other family members or close friends what they're worried about and what questions they have. Bring this list of questions to the appointment.
- Bring any required forms to your appointment. This

can include any medical paperwork requested and release from work forms for your employer.

- Keep a notebook with you at all appointments, phone calls and hospital visits, making notes of conversations you have with your surgeons, healthcare providers and insurance companies. Add any notes from messaging your physician offices via MyChart or other electronic medical record. Include contact information in this notebook.
- At the beginning of the appointment, tell your doctor that you have questions to ask. This will help the doctor set aside time to answer your questions. Try to ask your most important questions first.
- If you don't understand something, ask the doctor to explain it or to draw a picture. Keep these notes in your notebook or a special folder with all the patient's other medical information.
- If your first language is not English, interpreter services can be made available. Tell your doctor's office before your appointment if an interpreter is needed.
- If there's something you still don't understand when you get home, call the doctor's office or send a message through their online patient portal. Your doctor, a nurse navigator or other healthcare professional who works with the doctor may be able to answer many of your questions.

Questions You Might Ask Before Your Colon Resection Surgery Include:

- Why does my medical condition require colon resection surgery?
- Are there other treatment options? Why is this

surgery the preferred option?
- Are there other steps in the treatment and recovery process beyond the surgery itself?
- How comfortable and experienced are you with performing this type of surgery?
- Do you expect this to be a laparoscopic (done with smaller cuts) or open approach (done with a longer incision) to surgery? Why do you recommend that approach? What does this mean for me?
- Will I have any medication changes before or after surgery?
- Are there any tests or preoperative exams needed before surgery?
- How should I prepare for surgery?
- What are the main risks and complications of this procedure?
- What are the side effects of the colon resection? How can we manage them? Are these temporary or permanent?
- Are there any diet or lifestyle changes needed before or after surgery?
- When can I eat normal food?
- How will this surgery change how I eat or use the bathroom?
- Will I need an ostomy bag? If so, how can I and my caregiver get help or learn more?
- What can I expect while in the hospital?
- What can I expect the first week or two after surgery?
- When can I return to work? (Let your surgeon know what type of work you do; a more physical job may require a longer leave of absence or temporary adjustments to your job.)
- When can I expect to feel like my normal self?

- What strategies for comfort/pain reduction do you recommend?
- How should I reintroduce physical activity?
- When can I resume sexual activity?
- When should I contact the doctor or nurse? How do I contact them?

Bring Your Caregiver In Early

If you have a local support person such as a close friend, roommate or spouse who will assist you as a caregiver, see if they can go with you to all the appointments with the colon surgeon. If concerns or questions come up at home while you are recovering, your primary caregiver also can be the one to call the doctor. You should tell your healthcare provider to communicate with this person and include them on any release of information paperwork with the hospital and physician's office.

If you're the caregiver, it's important that you and the patient understand the planned colon surgery type, its possible side effects and what recovery is expected to look like. It's important to talk with the patient's healthcare providers and ask questions to help you understand how best to help the patient and when to seek out medical care after surgery.

Your caregiver can also be the main contact who shares updates about your recovery with family members and friends.

PREPARING FOR COLON SURGERY

Knowing you have a surgery coming up can be stressful. Beyond the medical preparation, there are logistical items for keeping "everything else" going during your surgery and recovery period. Here are actionable steps you can take to reduce stress as you prepare for the upcoming surgery.

Planning For Time Off At Work

It's not always easy to talk to your employer about needing surgery, but advance notice can go a long way. It allows your supervisor to find temporary resources to help cover your work and your teammates to plan for your time off. While you do not have to go into detail about your procedure, alert your employer to how long you anticipate being off work and what deadlines will occur during that time. What adjustments can be made to help your team out? Ask your coworkers if you can do anything to make this time go easier for them, particularly if they are picking up your workload while you're out. Keep your employer updated if your recovery changes and a return to work is delayed.

Remember that returning from a surgery is not like returning from a vacation. You will be away from the office for a longer period of time, and your body will take time to heal. Consider asking about remote or part-time options in your initial weeks back to work.

How Much Time Off To Plan For

Many patients, depending on the complexity of the surgery, can expect to spend two to seven days in the hospital, followed by a week or two at home in recovery before being cleared for light activity or driving.

For many people having a colon resection, they can return to work within six weeks. If your job is a more active one, such as driving all day, lifting objects, working outdoors or doing other physical work, or if you are receiving medical care for other health conditions, your recovery period may be longer. Always talk with your doctor about your time-off needs based on the physical requirements of your work, your recovery and any other health conditions you are living with. Don't be afraid to contact your doctor if you have concerns and may need to extend your time off work.

FMLA Basics

If you know in advance that you are needing colorectal surgery or you are caregiving for someone after surgery, follow your work's procedures and policies for applying for time off.

If you live in the United States, the Family and Medical Leave Act allows up to 12 weeks' time away from your work with job protection under certain conditions due to your or a family member's serious medical condition. You can take it in one block or several smaller blocks of time.

Do you qualify for FMLA? In general, private employers with at least 50 employees are covered by FMLA.

To qualify for FMLA:
- You must have worked for your employer for at least 12 months. Seasonal work does count.
- You must have worked for that employer for at least 1,250 hours in the 12 months before you take leave. That's an average of a little more than 24 hours a week, if you don't take other vacation time.
- You must work at a location where the employer has at least 50 employees within 75 miles of your worksite.
- You need to care for your spouse, child or parent who has a serious health condition, or you are unable to work because of your own serious health condition.

During your FMLA leave, you are allowed to keep your health insurance just as if you were not on leave during this time. Even if you are not getting paid, you can continue your insurance but may be required to continue to make any normal employee costs.

FMLA leave is unpaid leave, but sick time, vacation time or personal time can be used along with your FMLA leave so that you continue to get paid.

Private employers with fewer than 50 employees are not covered by the FMLA but may be covered by state family and medical leave laws.

When you return to work, FMLA requires that your employer return you to the same job that you left, or one that is nearly identical in duties, schedule or pay.

For more information on FMLA, read the Employee's Guide to the Family & Medical Leave Act, published by the United States Department of Labor.

For military families, read The Employee's Guide to Military Family Leave under the Family Medical Leave Act.

Caregiver Time Off

As the primary caregiver, you will want to make sure you plan for enough time off during the patient's recovery. If you are fortunate to know in advance about the procedure (versus an emergency surgery), work with your manager and team to create a plan for your time off.

Many surgeons state to plan for a hospital stay of typically up to seven days following a colectomy, and less if the surgery is done laparoscopically. But for some patients, complications can take place, resulting in a potential longer hospital stay or a delay in a return to normal activities. This can lead to a longer time away from work or other daily activities than initially planned.

HOUSEHOLD ORGANIZATION

Facing colon resection surgery can be daunting. Take the stress off you and your household during surgery week and the recovery period through simple steps toward household organization.

Finances

If you're receiving short-term disability or taking unpaid leave, you may need to readjust your budget during your recovery time and while you are recouping financially from increased expenses and decreased income. Nationally, 48 million Americans are unpaid caregivers, and three-fourths of family members are accruing thousands of dollars in out-of-pocket costs, including medical equipment, in-home care and office visits.

When first assessing your budget, estimate your temporary income, factoring in any short-term disability payments and out-of-pocket insurance expenses and known medical co-pays. Consider what regular expenses are needed (such as insurance, utilities, food, routine prescription medications and housing), what you can drop (gym fees, a sports session or subscriptions), and what you can get temporary assistance for through programs in your community or your network (such as meals). Create a temporary budget, with the goal to reassess after the first full month of income after resuming work.

Plan as much as you can for the unspoken expenses, such as lunch or dinner at the hospital for the caregiver (if you're there during meal time), additional over-the-counter supplies, gas, extra babysitters or after-school care, hospital parking and medications.

Contact your health insurance company to understand the details of your medical coverage and any copays or deductibles you may have. Many hospitals also offer payment plans to pay for medical expenses over time. Talk to the hospital's financial counselor or social worker to get started.

You may want to start a log of medical expenses, such as explanation of benefits received for medical services and the corresponding bills, to ensure all items are paid.

Meal Planning

Prepare extras of your family's favorite meals and freeze them. This can be accomplished in batch cooking, or just freezing single-serving packages of leftovers for the caregiver to use later.

Order some easy to prepare mini meals or snacks for your patient. Fast ideas that are shelf-stable include fruit cups, applesauce, instant mashed potatoes, and pudding cups.

Likewise, plan for simple, easy-to-prepare meals in your home for the rest of the family. Ideas can include grilled cheese and soup, pasta, heat-and-eat meals, cereals and muffins for breakfast, pre-cut vegetables and dips for snacks, and fresh fruit.

Patient Comfort

Prioritize rest and patient comfort to help you or your loved one be best able to recover after the procedure. Decide where your patient will sleep after they come home. Will it be in the bedroom? On the couch? Arm chair? Air mattress? Know where temporary sleeping arrangements will be for your patient, and for you as the caregiver, especially in those initial days when getting up and down is difficult.

If your shower or bedroom is located upstairs, you may want to consider temporarily moving sleeping and other accommodations downstairs, or limit reasons for your patient to come back downstairs once they are upstairs.

Clean your house before going to the hospital. Declutter major areas, such as the living room or bedroom where your patient will be spending more time in, as well as the hallways. If you're truly short on time, focus on the rooms and hallways where your patient is likely to be walking and the bathroom.

Group items you'll need in easy reach. This may be a small basket for medications that you'll be taking temporarily. Have a basket with "extras" for the bathroom, such as air freshener, wipes and extra toilet paper. Stage a phone or laptop charger or heating pad near your arm chair. Find an easy to reach shelf with snacks and disposable dishes and silverware for your patient.

The person who had surgery may need help with some activities of daily living, such as bathing, dressing or getting up and down from a chair or the toilet. Work with adult household members to make sure these needs are met.

Reduce Personal Stress At Home

Whether you are a patient or a caregiver, take whatever steps you can to reduce personal stress when you return from the hospital. This may include:

- Catch up on the laundry or any other routine chores.
- Recruit someone to walk the dog, mow the lawn, take out the trash or give kids a ride to school or activities. This can be a friend or teen or adult in the home who drives.
- Consider setting up grocery delivery if you don't utilize it already. This is particularly important as you will have driving and other physical restrictions after surgery.
- Clean out your car. Nothing is worse than worrying about tossing items into the backseat or shuffling trash on the car floor when you're already feeling sore.
- Refill any routine medications or medical supplies prior to your surgery.
- Fill up your gas tank on your vehicle.

Go Shopping

Buy some disposable dishes and silverware, including serving spoons. Save yourself from the dishes for one week. While you're at it, order extra toilet paper or flushable wipes. The early weeks will not be fun. Just have it delivered. Now is not the time to stress about not finding toilet paper on empty aisles in the grocery store.

Pick up any recommended over-the-counter medications or products before the surgery day.

Family Considerations

Depending on the age of the other members of your household, you may need to consider the following items:

Child Care

Plan for child care and assistance, even for evenings, morning prep and nights if you have a toddler or infant.

Household Tasks

Schedule your bill payments if they are not automatically submitted. Write on your calendar routine tasks such as trash collection for others who are assisting you.

Check Your Calendar

Check to see if any non-standard deadlines are looming. Is it time to renew your car tags? Is there a field trip coming up that needs a permission slip signed and money turned in? Is photo day at school looming? Order those photos online. Take advantage of online options such as gifts for birthdays - and pay for them to be wrapped and shipped. Order school supplies and Halloween costumes for delivery.

Daily Family Schedules

Plan for extra time for morning prep, after-school transitions, homework, dinner help, etc. You can say no to an extracurricular for a season while you're in recovery, or decline to participate in a school or church event. Energy focus should be on this season of recovery and maintaining some semblance of order at home, not taking on more tasks.

Contact Lists And Shared Calendar

Your caregiver should know who is taking family members where and when, as well as how to contact them in the event you are asleep or unable to assist.

School

Let your child's teacher know a surgery is coming up in case the child is acting out. Recruit a volunteer to help if your young child goes to a bus stop. If you're homeschooling, consider taking a few weeks off from homeschooling for surgery and recovery.

Preventing extra stress at home after the colectomy is important. Remember to be flexible and patient during the recovery process and this time of transition.

Recovery can take time, and it's important to prioritize the recovering patients' needs during this time. These simple steps can make the return home after colon surgery a much more manageable event.

TALKING TO YOUR KIDS ABOUT A COLECTOMY

Having a frank conversation with your family about what to expect while you're hospitalized and when you return home can reduce everyone's personal stress.

Prepare your kids. While you may be focused on your health, this surgery will have long-lasting challenges that will impact the children too. These range from financial (perhaps a temporary loss in income, or no funds for extracurricular activities) to transportation (relying on only one parent or a carpool to school or activities) to home life (parent in the recovery phase, which may or may not go quickly).

Children will quickly realize something is happening, and communicating in a sensitive, age-appropriate approach about your surgery and recovery is important. Remember, you set the stage for your child's reaction. If you are nervous, tense or upset about the surgery or underlying diagnosis, your child will pick up on these feelings.

Here are some of the topics you might cover:

What A Colectomy Is

Depending on the age and understanding of your children, the conversation you might have with them could be presented completely differently. One child may be curious to see pictures of the colonoscopy and learn all the particulars of the colon surgery. Another may simply need reassurance that dad would be okay.

For younger children, the language may be that "Mom is going to the hospital so the doctors can make her feel better, and she may be tired and sore for a few days after she returns home." Use age-appropriate language, such as "doctor" instead of "anesthesiologist." Reading books about going to the hospital can help as well.

Remind the child, this is temporary and it is part of making your parent healthy.

Discuss how home life will be impacted. Examples might include, "Dad is going to have surgery and it is going to be very busy while he gets better" or "Mrs. Smith is going to help us by taking you to school."

Household Tasks

Engage children and family members to assist around the house. Now is not the time for perfection, though you can take time before the surgery to introduce how to do new chores that will need to be done. You may use language like, "We need you to help out while dad is recovering. Can you help sweep the floor, vacuum and keep the bathroom clean for him for the next two weeks?"

For younger children, the message may be simpler: "Can you help bring mom water or a heating pad?" or "Can you reach the remote for her?"

Surgery Day And Hospitalization

Talk to your child about the day of surgery, any changes they can expect for that day and how they would feel better about the situation. Examples might be, "Would you like a text or email to the teacher when the surgery is over? It will be after lunch." or "Dad might not feel like talking after his surgery today, but would you like to text a silly picture after school?"

Activity After Returning Home

Explain in child-appropriate language how the patient will be impacted by the surgery.

Examples: "Dad cannot roughhouse and you cannot cuddle in his lap because he had surgery on his belly. But we can sit together while we watch a movie or read a favorite book." or "Mom can't play soccer at the park right now because she is getting better from surgery." Older children might hear: "We need your help to mow grass and take out the trash because mom has restrictions on how much she can lift."

Bathrooms

As hygiene habits may be impacted during your recovery, particularly in the early weeks, having a frank conversation with the kids about bathroom accessibility and habits is important.

Consider such statements as:

- "We need to keep the bathroom upstairs open in case mom needs it."
- "Yes, I know they feel like they're spending a lot of time in the bathroom."
- "Yes, the bathroom may smell different, please use some bathroom spray and don't make a big deal about it."
- "No, dad can't join us at the soccer game because there are no bathrooms. Right now he may need to use the restroom quickly."

Plan Something Special For The Kids

While this feels like one more thing to do, having an evening where you watch a favorite movie, bake cookies or eat pizza before the surgery or while one parent is in the hospital can make things feel a little more normal for your child.

COMMUNICATING WITH OTHER ADULTS

There may be people in your circle with whom you may share information about your upcoming surgery and recovery. Remember, as a patient, you are the one in control of what message(s) are shared. Additionally, you have control over who visits, and that can change throughout your healing journey.

Sharing Medical Matters

Decide in advance how much and how often you want to share updates on your colon surgery and recovery process.

- How will you spread the word - via a point person, CaringBridge, Facebook chat, text or email chain?
- Do you want to update individually or do group announcements?
- Do you want to limit communications to one update per day?
- Are there some people you don't want information given to?

- Are there some people whom you want to give more information to?
- Do you want to talk to your child's caregivers, teachers and other adults to let them know about surgery week? You may coordinate with teachers or daycare providers to extend the "Dad's OK" message on the day of the surgery to ease minds. Knowing that they may expect that message at a certain time can be beneficial.
- Do you want to be added to your church prayer chain or other unofficial support team?

Asking For Help

Often well-meaning people will offer a meal or to organize a meal train for your family during the initial period of hospitalization or after the return home. Here are some ways friends, coworkers and community members can help.

Meal Assistance

While many people do appreciate using meal scheduling sites like MealTrain or SignUpGenius, there are other ways that you can offer meal help for a family during and after a hospitalization. These include:

- Restaurant gift cards are great, but note that they can be difficult to use. Not all restaurants allow gift card redemption through their apps or websites, and coordinating time to drive to a restaurant, wait for preparation and return home may be difficult.

Instead, consider DoorDash, GrubHub or fast food gift cards, or offer meal cards for places that the caregiver can easily pick up on the way back from physician visits or the hospital.

- Gifts of paper plates, napkins and utensils
- Easy to prepare or grab-and-go breakfasts, particularly if work or school is still in session for family members
- Meals that are not frozen and can just be heated quickly. (Remembering to defrost items adequately in advance or timing the defrosting correctly can be a challenge at a time when schedules may be off.)
- Prepackaged snack items

Foods Specific To The Patient

The initial weeks after surgery will mean a more limited diet while the digestive system readjusts. Appreciated foods for a soft food diet can include:

- Soft foods such as applesauce or fruit cups, minute rice, tea, pasta, bananas, yogurt or pudding cups
- Pureed soups
- Boost or other protein drinks recommended by your surgery team
- Gatorade or other electrolyte drinks due to the risk of dehydration

Comfort Gifts

Comfort gifts for patients can include:

- Soft blanket
- Books by favorite authors (print or e-book)
- Magazines
- Loose-fitting pajamas
- Soups
- Warm socks or slippers
- Lotion

Household Help

Helping the household run more smoothly is very much appreciated during a caregiving phase. This might include:

- Rides or carpools to school or extracurricular activities
- Play dates
- Mowing the lawn or weeding
- Pet care
- Small chores around the house
- Offering gas cards due to the extra driving to physician visits and hospitals
- Lunch pickup from summer free lunch programs
- Additional packages of toilet paper

Taking time to discuss needs with family, loved ones and friends can help reduce frustrations during the weeks after surgery.

SURGERY AND HOSPITALIZATION

Your preparation for colon surgery can actually begin a few weeks before the event.

Easing Into Surgery

After learning about the need for surgery, you may be scheduled for a preoperative physical to make sure you're at your healthiest before surgery. Your pre-op appointment is a great time to discuss any concerns, such as pain control and what has worked or not worked for you in the past. Your doctor may ask you to stop smoking if you smoke and stop taking certain medications such as blood thinners for a period of time.

You'll also want to take steps to prevent potential exposure to viruses such as COVID-19 and flu viruses. Being sick can potentially cause your surgery to be postponed.

Advance Directives

While no one wants to think things can go wrong during or after surgery, complications can happen. Writing or updating your advance directive can put your caregiver, spouse or healthcare proxy at ease about what medical decisions to make if you were unable to speak for yourself.

Laws about advance directives vary by state. You can download state-specific advance directive forms from your state government website. Complete your advance directives, give a copy to your healthcare representative, and make sure your physician and hospital have a copy.

Types of advance directives include:

Living Will

A living will is a written, legal document that describes the medical treatments you would want or not want if you were terminally ill or permanently unconscious.

Physician Order For Life-Sustaining Treatment

A physician order for life-sustaining treatment, or POLST, is for people who have been diagnosed with a serious illness. A POLST is filled out by your doctor but doesn't replace your other advance directives.

Durable Power Of Attorney For Healthcare

A durable power of attorney or medical power of attorney states which person you have chosen to be a healthcare proxy make medical decisions for you. It becomes active any time you are unconscious or unable to make medical decisions for yourself. While you may be married and feel you do not need a healthcare proxy, the reality is family battles can and do occur over medical care. A medical power of attorney is not the same as a financial power of attorney.

Do Not Resuscitate

A do-not-resuscitate (DNR) order can also be part of an advance directive but can be a separate document. This tells hospital staff that if CPR would be needed that you don't want to be resuscitated if your breathing or heart stops.

Colon Surgery Preparations

Within the week or two of your surgery date, you may be asked to stop certain prescription medications and over-the-counter products such as aspirin, Advil, Motrin, ibuprofen, Aleve, naproxen, fish oil, vitamins and herbal supplements. These may increase your risk of bleeding during or after surgery.

If you smoke tobacco or use marijuana in any form, your physician may ask you to stop that as well. Smoking can put you at a higher risk of complications after surgery, including pneumonia, heart attacks and infections. Marijuana use, including edibles, can impact how your body reacts to anesthesia.

A day or two before your colon prep for surgery, begin switching to lower-fiber foods. Your surgeon may ask you to limit certain foods, such as corn.

Day Before Surgery

The day before surgery, you'll begin colon prep, much like if you were having a colonoscopy. Your day may start with a very limited diet (like toast or hard boiled eggs) then progress to a clear liquid diet. It's a great day for the rest of the household to enjoy those meals you hate but they love.

As the day progresses, you will switch to a combination of a large bottle of laxative diluted with Gatorade or other clear liquid. Plan for a long day and longer night. Be prepared for an uncomfortable night for everyone; in fact, the caregiver might consider sleeping in another bedroom if they can, simply because of the waking up and down. That way, the caregiver can be well-rested.

The night before and day of surgery, follow your surgeon's instructions regarding fluids, eating, bathing with antibacterial soap and other steps.

You may be asked to take antibiotics for a few days to prevent infection.

Surgery Day Tips For The Family

- Family members should prepare for your time during the procedure. Plan on at least half a day in the surgery waiting room. How will you spend it? Leave and return, or stay? Do you prefer to work remotely on "busy work" that requires little mental effort vs. attending meetings or staring at the waiting room's TV screen all day?
- If you stay in the surgery waiting room, bring something relaxing to read or do to pass the time.
- Bring a notebook to take notes of things that need to get done or notes from the surgeon and medical staff.
- Call or text friends. (And it is OK to just forward a response to any questions, delay in responding or state that you'll update everyone at a certain time.)
- Today's the day to splurge on that favorite coffee drink or a nice lunch, even if your heart doesn't feel like it.
- Take time for you. Walk, drive the kids to school, or just step out of the hospital waiting room for a moment if you need to. Simply let the waiting room staff know what phone number to reach you at.

What To Bring To The Hospital

Your caregiver can bring a bag of personal items to your patient room after you are settled after surgery.

Consider packing:

- Cell phone or tablet
- Extra long cord for phone

- Reading material
- Notebook and pen
- Underwear and loose clothing to wear at the hospital if you prefer not to wear a hospital gown
- Unscented deodorant
- Loose-fitting clothes for going home
- Slip-on shoes for going home
- Baby wipes or face wipes for feeling fresh in the hospital, especially if showering is not an option yet
- Brush or comb
- Glasses, hearing aids and dentures
- Toiletries such as toothbrushes etc.
- You may be asked to bring your inhaler or eye drops, however most medications will be dispensed by the hospital pharmacy while you are there.

Leave your wallet, medications, jewelry and wedding ring at home.

Tips For Your Hospital Stay

- Talk with the surgeon and other members of the healthcare team about any questions you have.
- Your doctor may have you wear support stockings or air sleeves to help the circulation in your legs while being in bed. This is to help prevent blood clots.
- You will learn to use a small machine called a spirometer for deep breathing exercises. This will help reduce your chances of developing pneumonia after surgery.
- Resist the urge to "tough out" pain. If your doctor says pain medication is to be taken only when needed,

request it when you are beginning to feel pain. It will take time for the medication to arrive on the unit, and the stronger the pain level is, the more difficult it is to bring it back under control.

- Use a nurse call light while in pain. Also alert your care team if you have any discomfort such as rash, itching or swelling.
- During flu season and the coronavirus pandemic, the numbers of daily visitors have been often restricted; consider a video chat or phone call instead if you want to catch up. It's also OK to decline visitors, or delay a response to a text or call if you don't feel up to visiting with others.
- If children are not allowed to visit, plan a daily video chat or call, watch TV together on the phone or play an online game together.
- You will ease into activity, such as sitting up in your bed or moving to a chair. A physical therapist may visit you to give you exercises and help you progress to walking. Caregivers can help support their patient by walking with them, encouraging them with breathing exercises and rehab exercises.
- When you are ready to go home, medical staff will review your care plan and any scheduled follow-up appointments. Inquire about whether home health services may be needed, even if for one or two consultations at home.

RECOVERING FROM A COLECTOMY

You may have big goals for once you "feel better" colon resection after surgery, but your body may have other plans.

Remember that you just had surgery, and your surgery recovery and feelings of tiredness may continue for several weeks. Give yourself grace if you can't immediately do everything you want.

For the greatest success, follow your doctor's after-care instructions. They may be printed on an after-visit summary packet given to you at the doctor's office or hospital, a patient handout, or pre-surgical education. Your future you depends on the choices you make today.

Caring For Your Loved One After A Colectomy

Caring for your loved one in the early days after a colectomy can be a daunting task, particularly if they have not been eating solid foods much. It's OK for caregivers to be nervous if you have never cared for someone after a surgery before. Caregivers do take on a large amount of responsibility, from the day-to-day care and the "what if's."

Respect your patient's needs and help your loved one balance recovery with a growing desire for independence.

Tips for helping your loved one with recovery include:

- Encourage them to continue breathing exercises as directed by their physician. Breathing exercises help you to clear your lungs and reduce your risk of developing pneumonia in the days after surgery.
- Keep the pain medication on schedule as prescribed in the initial days. Don't wait until the pain becomes unmanageable and you're having to chase it to get the pain levels down.
- Take brief walks. These walks may be shorter walks than you are typically used to. They may be as simple as walking to the mailbox or corner.
- Use comfort measures such as sitting in a recliner or using a heating pad.
- Respect whether your loved one wants visitors in the home while in recovery. Realize this may change hour to hour.
- Remind your loved one they don't have to answer every call and can put their phone on silent when they are feeling less talkative. Calls and messages can be returned.

Talk with the surgeon and other members of the healthcare team about any questions you have, even once your loved one is out of the hospital. Often you can send messages online through MyChart or other electronic health records system, or you can place a phone call.

Reasons to call your doctor or seek immediate medical care after colon resection surgery include:

- Pain that does not get better after you take pain medicine
- Not being able to have bowel movements or pass gas for more than 24 hours, or within the timeframe your physician advises
- Nausea or vomiting; being unable to keep fluids down
- Not able to take anything solid or liquid by mouth for 24 hours
- Abdominal swelling or pain
- Bright red blood has soaked through the bandage
- Loose stitches
- The incision comes open.
- Fever
- Pain in the calf, back of the knee, thigh or groin. These are signs of a potential blood clot in the leg.
- Redness and swelling in the leg or groin
- Increased pain, swelling, warmth or redness
- Red streaks leading from the incision
- Pus draining from the incision, which can be a sign of infection
- High ostomy output
- Dark urine or no urine

Go to the emergency room if you have chest pain or shortness of breath.

Sleep

Before you go to the hospital, you should discuss options for sleeping arrangements for after your return home.

A spouse or significant other might not consider sleeping arrangements at home in the initial weeks after their surgery. Much like with a c-section, abdominal pain can be a very real reality during the initial recovery period following a colectomy. A person who tosses and turns in their sleep or sleeps with their body overlapping the other person may need to consider sleeping on a sofa or air mattress during the initial healing period. Remember also that what was once a comfortable sleep position may no longer be comfortable in the early days and weeks after surgery. Consider laying on your back with your head propped up with pillows, placing pillows in strategic positions to ease discomfort, or sleeping in an armchair.

The caregiver who will be assisting at night also needs to consider where they will be sleeping. Getting up and down throughout the night to assist with medications, going to the bathroom or other helping your patient become more comfortable may be part of your initial return home, so plan where the caregiver sleeps accordingly.

Tips for getting a good night's sleep for both patients and caregivers include:

- Have a regular sleep routine.
- Get some form of exercise or stress reduction daily.
- Cut down on caffeine.
- Reduce lights in your room to create a darkened space.

- Remove distractions.
- Keep a notepad on your bed to jot down any thoughts you need to act on later.

Pain Management

While your surgeon will work with you on pain control in the initial period after surgery, you'll likely have some temporary help in the form of prescription or over-the-counter medications such as ibuprofen or Aleve to help reduce inflammation. If you are on Norco, do not take Tylenol, as both medications have acetaminophen, and too much acetaminophen can be hard on your liver.

Since you've had surgery in your abdominal area, you'll want to splint the area by holding a pillow against it while coughing or deep breathing.

Be sure to talk to your doctor if the pain does not go away in the recovery process or gets worse over time. Other pain relief options such as a nerve block may ultimately be considered if other measures do not work to relieve pain.

Non-prescription ways to help reduce pain include heating pads, lidocaine patches, distraction with music, favorite shows or podcasts, and guided imagery. Finding creative outlets such as music or art have been shown to reduce depression, pain and tiredness and improve immune function.

Passing The Time

Recovering from a colectomy can take weeks or months, and previous hobbies and activities may not be an option for some time. You may have pain, complications, or an ostomy bag to contend with.

Here are ideas to pass the time while recovering from colon surgery:

- Read that novel you've been meaning to read.
- Write in a journal.
- Learn stress-reducing techniques like meditation, visualization or contemplative prayer.
- Organize your photos.
- Plan an outing or day trip (or go bigger!) for when you've fully recovered.
- Plan next year's garden.
- Create a Pinterest board for that next house project.
- Plan those home projects and recruit help.
- Meal prep for when you return to work or regular activities.
- Write thank you notes to those who helped.
- Volunteer from home. Sites such as VolunteerMatch, Points of Light, DoSomething.org, GiveGab and Encoure.org can offer ideas for remote volunteer work.
- Learn a new skill online.
- Update your LinkedIn profile or resume.
- Discover a new podcast.

Exercise

Daily physical activity - everything from stretching to walking - helps your body with the digestion process and helps prevent buildup of intestinal gas and constipation. Try to walk each day. Start by walking a little more than you did the day before. Bit by bit, increase the amount you walk, building up to 30 minutes or more most days of the week.

Walking provides additional benefits for surgery recovery, as it boosts blood flow and helps prevent pneumonia and constipation.

Avoid strenuous activities, such as biking, jogging, weight lifting or aerobic exercise, until your doctor says.

Avoid lifting anything that would make you strain until your doctor gives you permission. This may include heavy grocery bags, milk jugs, a heavy briefcase or backpack, cat litter or dog food bags, a vacuum cleaner or a child.

Driving

Driving is not recommended for at least two weeks after your colon surgery and until you have stopped taking narcotic pain medications. However you may find that while you're cleared to drive, you may have stiffness or soreness while driving a vehicle, particularly when turning or making quick movements. Ease into driving, and start with a brief drive around your block at a quiet time of day to test how you feel.

Bowel Movements

Particularly in the first few weeks after colon resection, you'll likely experience more frequent, looser bowel movements than you did before the surgery. Be sure that you're drinking adequate fluids to prevent dehydration.

To prevent constipation, make sure to eat adequate fiber, continue physical activity, drink liquids and don't ignore the urge to go. Fiber supplements, laxatives or stool softeners can be used if your physician recommends it.

To prevent diarrhea, limit high-fat foods and choose more plant-based foods, which can contain more fiber. Additionally, limit caffeinated, carbonated and alcoholic beverages, all of which can irritate the stomach.

From a personal comfort standpoint, invest in extra toilet paper or wipes, and consider an air freshener, scented candle or diffuser in your bathrooms to reduce potential embarrassment.

Ostomy

Some people will require an ostomy bag to remove their waste from their bodies after their colon resection surgeries. While it sounds rare, about 1 million people are currently living with an ostomy, according to the United Ostomy Associations of America.

Instead of having a regular bowel movement, a colostomy bag is attached to the stoma, or opening, on your abdomen.

These bags may be a closed bag that needs changing multiple times a day or drainable bags that need to be replaced every few days. Colostomy bags have air filters with charcoal that can work to neutralize the smell.

Other options include irrigation, or using an enema in your stoma to rinse your bowels. This is an hour-long task that requires a routine time commitment each day.

A nurse specializing in stoma care can help train you on the proper use of your colostomy supplies. You may learn about this in the hospital, in the outpatient setting or in home care.

You will be able to do most forms of exercise with a stoma, and you can travel and continue to work at most jobs without issue.

Living With Short Bowel Syndrome

After a colon resection, particularly one that removes a large portion of your colon, you may be living with short bowel syndrome. Short bowel syndrome is when your remaining bowel adapts after surgery and cannot absorb enough nutrients and fluids, leading to various health complications.

These recurring symptoms can include:

- Abdominal pain
- Anemia
- Bloating
- Cramping
- Dehydration
- Diarrhea

- Fatigue
- Food sensitivity
- Gas
- Heartburn
- Weakness
- Weight loss.

Complications from short bowel syndrome can include malnutrition, kidney stones, peptic ulcers and bacterial overgrowth in the intestine.

Short bowel syndrome impacts about three out of every 1 million people. There is no cure for short bowel syndrome, but with medication management and lifestyle changes, you can manage many of its symptoms.

If you have short bowel syndrome, experts suggest these tips to ease discomfort:

- Eat more frequent, smaller meals that are easier to digest.
- Consider drinking liquids between meals instead of during meals.
- Eat more protein.
- Choose complex carbohydrates instead of simple sugars, which can cause diarrhea.
- Take a multivitamin each day. Many people with short bowel syndrome have difficulties absorbing nutrients into their diet.
- Limit your alcohol and caffeine intake.

Living with short bowel syndrome can be physically uncomfortable for the patient and may require changes for the family. This may mean having a bathroom available for the patient, particularly in the initial weeks after colon resection surgery, planning ahead that the other adult in the home is on call for rides for children to activities, and delays or changes to family activities that were once routine.

For some people, short bowel syndrome will be a temporary problem lasting the first year or two after surgery while your body adjusts to having a shortened intestinal tract. For others, nutritional support, IV feeding, supplements, bowel transplant or other surgery may be needed as part of their long-term care plan.

While short bowel syndrome is a chronic condition that doesn't go away on its own, with proper treatment and management, many people with short bowel syndrome can lead full and healthy lives.

Small Bowel Obstruction

A small bowel obstruction is a possible complication that requires medical attention. This is when a blockage in your bowels prevents contents from moving through your intestines. Signs are abdominal pain or distention, vomiting of fecal matter, and constipation.

DIET CHANGES AFTER COLON RESECTION SURGERY

After colon resection surgery, your gastrointestinal system has changed. Your diet will too as it adjusts to the changes from colon surgery.

Soft Food Diet After Colectomy

Your doctor will likely prescribe a soft food diet for the first initial weeks as you recover from your colon resection. Think of soft, moist foods like soups, gelatin, pudding and yogurt.

As you progress to being able to eat and tolerate more solid foods, take small bites and choose your food well. Reintroduce foods slowly and be aware of any effects, and know that each body is different. Even a simple grilled cheese sandwich could cause distress for some people. Introduce new foods in small amounts, and if you experience discomfort, you might wait to try again until after further healing.

Remember, the way your foods are prepared can make a difference in how your body handles them. Raw vegetables, for example, are discouraged after a colon resection surgery as they may cause gas. Steaming or microwaving vegetables helps to preserve nutrients. Consider using a blender for smoothies, soups or purees. Avoid initially tough meats, spicy, and fried foods.

Avoid any foods that you know cause stomach gas and distention, including corn, beans, peas, lentils, onions, broccoli, cauliflower and cabbage.

Foods To Avoid Initially After Colon Resection Surgery

After your colon resection, certain foods and drinks will be discouraged by your doctor in the initial weeks while your body adjusts to life with a smaller colon.

Avoid these types of foods in the initial weeks after your colectomy:

- Raw fruits and vegetables
- Tough meats such as beef or pork
- Whole grain, multi-grain, chewy or crispy breads
- High-fiber foods
- Nuts and seeds
- Fried, greasy foods
- Spicy foods

Beverages

Beverages to avoid:
- Carbonated drinks
- Alcohol
- Citrus juices
- Chocolate drinks
- Caffeinated drinks
- Coffee

Choose these beverages instead:
- Milk (animal or plant-based)
- Decaf tea
- Powdered drink mixes
- Non-citrus juices
- Water

Grains

Grains to avoid:
- Whole-grain breads and cereals
- Anything with seeds, nuts, raisins, dried fruit or coconut
- Whole-grain rice
- Sweet rolls, coffee cake, donuts
- Seasoned crackers
- Popcorn

Choose these grains instead:
- Ready-to-eat cereal
- Refined bread
- Crackers such as saltines

- Plain white rice
- White pasta
- Pancakes and waffles

Protein

Protein sources to avoid:
- Anything fried
- Tough meats with gristle
- Smoked meats
- Sausage
- Shellfish
- Fatty meats
- Cold cuts/lunch meat
- Fried eggs
- Dried beans
- Nuts and seeds
- Crunchy peanut butter

Choose these protein sources:
- Tender meat, pork, poultry and fish, prepared baked, broiled, boiled, roasted, stewed or simmered
- Eggs
- Tofu
- Creamy peanut butter

Dairy

Dairy products to avoid:
- Sharp/strong cheeses
- Dairy with nuts or seeds
- Cheese with peppers

Choose these dairy products:
- Low-fat milk products
- Smooth yogurt
- Mild cheese
- Cottage cheese

Vegetables

Avoid these vegetables:
- Raw vegetables
- Broccoli
- Brussels sprouts
- Cabbage
- Onions
- Cauliflower
- Corn
- Cucumber
- Dried beans, peas, and lentils
- Fried potatoes or potato chips
- Green peppers
- Radishes
- Sauerkraut
- Tomatoes, tomato sauce

Choose these vegetables:
- Soft-cooked or canned vegetables
- Fresh lettuce and tomato
- Potatoes without the skin (boiled, mashed, baked or creamed)

Fruit

Avoid these fruits:
- Dried fruits
- Fruits with skins, seeds or pits, such as berries, figs or raisins
- All citrus fruits and juices
- Ripe bananas
- Coconut

Choose these fruits:

- Most soft, raw fruits (eaten without skin)
- Cooked and canned fruits
- Fruit juice

Fats and Sweets

Avoid these fats and sweets:
- Spicy salad dressings
- Bacon or bacon fat
- Lard
- Salt pork
- Fried foods
- Nuts
- Any foods with dried fruit, nuts, coconut, candied fruit
- Crunchy peanut butter
- Peanut brittle
- Sugar substitutes like sorbitol, xylitol, erythritol or sorbitol

Enjoy these fats and sweets in moderation:
- Ice cream, sherbet and frozen yogurt
- Pudding
- Cake
- Cookies without hard pieces
- Sugar
- Syrup
- Honey
- Jelly
- Seedless jam
- Butter and margarine
- Mayonnaise and vegetable oils
- Mildly seasoned salad dressings and sauces
- Plain, low-fat cream cheese
- Low-fat sour cream

Probiotics And Prebiotics

With probiotics and prebiotics, enjoy them as nature intended: within the food itself instead of taking supplements, unless your surgeon recommends them. Supplements are generally regarded as safe, but the American Gastroenterology Association says there may be no real benefit in ingesting probiotic supplements for gut health.

Probiotics are active, live cultures that aid in digestion. Foods including probiotics include:
- Buttermilk
- Fermented vegetables
- Kimchi
- Kombucha

- Miso
- Pickles
- Sauerkraut
- Sourdough
- Tempeh
- Yogurt

Prebiotics are the components in food that help feed probiotics. They can reduce symptoms of irritable bowel syndrome or diarrhea. Foods including prebiotics include:

- Fruits and vegetables
- Grains
- Legumes
- Oats

Meal Planning

The initial weeks after surgery can feel overwhelming to plan for meals for the patient and for the rest of the family. They might not be up for the same foods you are, and some days they may not be physically ready to eat at your usual mealtime. Instead, consider a routine of meals for the rest of the family and the patient eating what and when they can.

Meals to consider for the whole family:

- Soup
- Pasta (no heavy sauces or cheeses)
- Chicken (no skin)
- Grilled cheese sandwiches
- Rice dishes

Consider also bolstering a main dish everyone can eat with sides for the hungrier family members.

As your family member returns to more normal eating, you may find common foods may no longer be in the mix, nor as frequently.

MENTAL HEALTH AFTER SURGERY

Taking care of one's mental health is essential. During this season of recovery, you may run through crisis/fight-or-flight mode, then ease into chronic stress that may ebb and flow, but stress from the effects of surgery may remain present in some form.

Going through a surgery as a family feels personal, but it's not. Surgery just is, and your attitude can shape the healing process for your family.

Mental Health And Your Recovery

You may have heard your mental and physical health are related, but it's important to your recovery after colon surgery. Psychological stress can cause an inflammatory response in your body, which can slow recovery.

After surgery, you may experience feelings of loneliness, frustration with your progress, anger or irritation. Additionally, being in pain or being tired can erode your mental defenses.

Researchers have found a link between pain and feelings of depression and anxiety, particularly when dealing with chronic pain. If these feelings persist for more than two weeks, speak to your physician. Depression and anxiety can occur up to one year after surgery.

To help alleviate these feelings, care for your mental health. Build a routine of getting out of bed and dressing each day, reach out to others, go outside, exercise, eat a healthy diet, and work towards a sleeping schedule. Divide things into "I can," "I should" and "I must" - and prioritize accordingly.

Talk to your friends, family or therapist if you feel overwhelmed by emotions. You may also find support groups helpful to know you aren't alone in these life changes.

Try to focus on positive aspects in life, even if they seem small. Gratitude can improve your mental health and help you feel more hopeful for the future.

Remember, recovery is a journey. It's essential to be patient and kind to yourself as you navigate this new chapter in your life. Give yourself time to adjust. Don't rush the healing process or put pressure on yourself to be back to your old routine quickly.

Caregiver Stress

In the days after returning home from colon surgery, you may be spending more time assisting with moving around, including getting up and down from chairs or toilets, helping with pain management, getting items and helping your patient become more comfortable physically. That, combined with reduced or interrupted sleep, can lead to an increase in physical and mental stress.

In the days and first weeks after colon surgery, you may be reluctant to leave your patient to use some of your more typical stress-relieving activities, such as going to the gym, running outside or taking a long bath.

Instead, look for small ways to encourage stress-reduction in your home and your lifestyle. This may include working remotely, working reduced hours or taking time off work, planning for grab-and-go snacks and meals, and napping when the patient is.

But caregiver stress doesn't just happen in the initial weeks after surgery. The ongoing changes in lifestyle impacts the rest of the household, too. Caring for a loved one who has gone through a life-changing surgery can be physically and mentally draining. It's important for caregivers to take care of their own physical and mental health during this time and to avoid burnout and ensure you are able to provide the best possible care for your loved one.

Signs Of Caregiver Stress

Signs of caregiver stress can include:

- Feeling overwhelmed
- Feeling alone, isolated, or deserted by others
- Sleeping too much or too little
- Gaining or losing a lot of weight
- Feeling tired most of the time
- Losing interest in activities you used to enjoy

- Becoming easily irritated or angered
- Feeling worried or sad often
- Having headaches or body aches often
- Feeling constantly worried
- Abusing alcohol or drugs, including prescription medications

Reducing Your Stress

You have tools to help reduce your stress as a caregiver. Among the tips to cut caregiver stress:

- Recognize you're in a time of change, and that surgery recovery is temporary.
- Realize what you can and cannot control. Identify one thing you can change that can reduce your stress. It can be as simple as having paper plates and disposable silverware for a week, so you don't have to do battles with the children over the dishes.
- Focus on what you can do. Keep a "got done" list. Knowing you got the dishes done, a few bills paid and a load of laundry started can offer a huge mental relief that progress was being made.
- Prioritize what must be done. Note deadlines for time-sensitive items, from bills to permission slips. Consider pausing some volunteer efforts during this time. Consider telling groups you are involved with that you will not be attending meetings, but may be available over email and could help with some small, specific tasks that you could do from home.
- Accept help from friends, Meals on Wheels, or local transportation services. If you're unsure, ask about agencies that could provide care.
- Set clear boundaries. That can include: "I need to set

time to exercise" or "I cannot help with the PTA event this year." No need to apologize.

- Find a social outlet. Join a walking buddy once a week, find a person you can talk to or text when needed, attend an in-person or virtual Bible study, or grab a coffee with a colleague.
- Disconnect when you need to. Watching everyone live life while you are at home caring for someone can feel disheartening and make you feel forgotten. Caregivers who use social media more often report feeling alone, according to the AARP. Logging off social media and the stream of photos of others fully living their lives can make a huge difference in your mental health.
- Find support. You can find in-person and online support groups related to conditions such as colon cancer or irritable bowel syndrome. Talking with others going through similar experiences can reduce feelings of isolation and provide emotional support.
- Practice stress reduction. Walk, stretch or find short videos or apps online.
- Set a goal of one thing you'd like to accomplish in three to six months.
- Notice the positive things in your life, and share the news. Start a gratitude journal or posting each day.
- List your annoyances; you may realize that they are truly quite small.
- Have a daily routine, even if it's simple in the beginning, like wake up and shower.
- Take breaks. Caregiving can be a 24/7 job early in the recovery process but it's important for you to take breaks and prioritize your self care. That can include walking, relaxing, or participating in a favorite hobby. It also means caring for yourself physically, including

getting enough sleep, proper hydration, exercise and eating regular meals and maintaining your health. If it all feels overwhelming, talk to your doctor.

- Practice self-compassion. Caregiving can be challenging and emotionally draining, but it's important to be kind to yourself and practice self-compassion. Remember you are doing the best you can under circumstances not many people can understand.

Long-term stress of any kind can impact your physical and mental health, including:

- Anxiety
- Arthritis
- Cancer
- Depression
- Diabetes
- Heart disease
- High blood pressure
- Short-term memory problems

You can take a short caregiver self-assessment questionnaire from the American Medical Association to help evaluate your well-being. The link is in the sources section at the back of this book.

If you are struggling with mental health, it's important to seek professional support. A therapist or counselor can provide support and help you develop coping strategies to manage the challenge of caregiving. And, if it truly feels too much and you are considering self-harm or suicide, call or text 988.

Temporary Feelings and Emotions

Remember that it's OK to have days when the negative emotions come up. It's perfectly OK to say you are overwhelmed, don't want to do this any longer, wish this season in life was over. It is OK to say when you feel like things are hopeless and you have no control over the healing process. It is OK to say you were angry and frustrated, that you're tired of the slow progress, that you're annoyed with the person you're caring for. It's OK to be annoyed with caregiving. It's OK to say you feel things are out of control.

It is OK. Feelings are part of being human.You might be grieving your old lifestyle. You might even feel guilty for having those feelings. Acknowledge your feelings, and be sure to share them: journal, join a support community, talk with a professional, call or text a close friend or family member. Not giving your feelings air can lead to you coping poorly or engaging in unhealthy habits.

When you're overwhelmed and overloaded with emotion, remember to slow down, breathe, pray, meditate, do what you need to take a break from the moment.

Caregiver Depression

According to the Family Caregiver Alliance, more than 20 percent of family caregivers suffer from depression.

These signs may indicate depression:
- Agitation
- Anxiety

- Apathy
- Excessive crying
- Excessive hunger or loss of appetite
- Fatigue
- Feelings of hopelessness
- Insomnia
- Irritability
- Loss of interest or pleasure in activities
- Mood swings
- Restlessness
- Sadness
- Social isolation
- Thoughts of suicide
- Too much sleep
- Unable to concentrate
- Weight gain or weight loss

It is important for family caregivers to recognize and address signs of depression, as it can affect their ability to provide care and impact their overall well-being. Seeking help and support is the first step in managing depression and improving mental health. Talk to your healthcare professional, such as their primary care physician or a mental health provider, to get an assessment of their symptoms and receive appropriate treatment. If you are considering harming yourself or have thoughts of suicide, call 988, the National Suicide Prevention Lifeline.

Loneliness

One in five caregivers say they feel alone, and that number is even higher when one is caring for their spouse, according to the AARP. That feeling of loneliness is linked to increased stress and decreased physical health.

As a caregiver, it can be challenging to find time to get out and connect with other people. However, it's important to make time for social connections to prevent feelings of isolation and loneliness. Here are some ways caregivers can get out and connect with other people:

- Attend support groups: Join a support group for caregivers in your area. This is a great way to meet other caregivers who understand what you're going through and can offer support and advice.
- Volunteer: Volunteering is a great way to get out and meet new people. Look for volunteer opportunities in your community that align with your interests. Some volunteer opportunities may be for a single day or afternoon, others may be for a more extended period of time.
- Join a club or group: Join a club or group that interests you, such as a book club, knitting group or sports team. This is a great way to meet new people who share your interests.
- Take a class: Sign up for a class in something you've always wanted to learn, such as cooking, painting, or dancing. This is a great way to meet new people and learn a new skill.
- Attend events: Attend local events in your community, such as fairs, festivals, or concerts. This is a great way to get out and meet new people while also enjoying some entertainment.

If you're concerned about getting outside of the home and leaving your loved one alone, look for a friend to accompany them for a few hours while you get outside.

Remember, it's important to take care of yourself as a caregiver, and that includes making time for social connections. By connecting with others, you can reduce feelings of isolation and loneliness, and also gain support and encouragement.

Balancing Work And Caregiving

More than 60 percent of caregivers are balancing work and caregiving, according to AARP Public Policy Institute. On the average, these caregivers are working nearly 40 hours a week - on top of their personal responsibilities and caregiving. As a result, many are working adjusted hours, taking leaves of absence, turning down promotions, or receiving warnings about performance or attendance. Not surprising, of these employees, more than 60 percent say caregiving impacts their job.

If you're a caregiver, be transparent about your caregiving situation with your supervisor, take advantage of FMLA if needed, and utilize your local employee assistance program for emotional support. If you're able, inquire into remote work, flexible schedules, eldercare referrals and resources such as respite care as well.

Be sure to set realistic expectations about what you can achieve in a day. We are all gifted with the same 24 hours, and you can only do so much with that time. Make a list of the most important tasks that need to be done and prioritize them, allowing for time for the unexpected to occur. Don't overcommit yourself and set yourself up for failure.

To help stay organized, keep track of appointments, tasks and deadlines with a shared calendar or planner. This can help you stay on top of things and avoid feeling overwhelmed.

It's easy to get overwhelmed and stressed when balancing work and caregiving responsibilities. Try to stay positive and focus on the things that you are able to accomplish. Remember to celebrate small victories and take pride in your accomplishments.

Caring For Your Mental And Physical Health

While you are caring for a loved one, be sure to take the time to schedule your health needs, too. Your schedule may be different, from running to the hospital for visiting hours, up in the middle of the night to assist the patient, or filling in on errands or household responsibilities. But caring for yourself is one of the most important (and often forgotten) things you need to do as a caregiver.

According to the Family Caregiver Alliance, family caregivers - regardless of age - are less likely than their peers to do self care and preventive health steps. Among their challenges:

- Eating healthfully
- Exercising consistently
- Making medical appointments for themselves
- Getting enough sleep
- Resting when ill

Additionally, caregivers are more likely than non-caregivers to have chronic medical conditions such as high blood pressure, high cholesterol and being overweight. Talk to your doctor if you are struggling with your medical conditions, stress levels, sleep or healthy habits during this time. Your doctor may have alternate solutions for you to consider and can be a support person on your team.

Personal health setbacks are not a time saver. Schedule that time for a walk. Take your medicine. Drink your water. Eat a healthy meal. Take a nap. Make you a priority, even for small moments.

ACTIVE LIVING AFTER COLON RESECTION SURGERY

You may have been cleared to work, exercise or drive. But a return to a life completely like the one you lived before your colon surgery may not fully be an option. Digestive habits, tiredness, pain, or mental health may still have a lingering impact on your daily life. But you can still return to an active lifestyle with a little planning.

Changing Needs And Keeping The Pace

As your surgery recovery continues from weeks to months, you may find yourself evolving from requiring day-to-day medical support to needing assistance with getting on track with household activities. Recovery doesn't stop once a return to normal activity begins, and you may find yourself tiring more than you used to as your body spends its energy recovering.

When you have recovered enough to be cleared by your doctor to return to the workplace, the workday itself and commute may be enough to tire you out. This may mean there are holes that need to be filled: the chores, the homework battles, running errands and picking up kids.

The return to work is a great time to invest in shortcuts to make things a bit easier. You might save the gift cards you'd gotten during the surgery - which would have meant extra trips out during a challenging home time - for easy dinners to pick up after work. Plan meals, invest in grocery delivery and look at bundling your pharmacy pickups. Sit down as a family each Sunday to review the week ahead.

Workplace Accommodations

Most people can return to work after colon resection surgery, however, some people experiencing bowel changes may need accommodations at work. If you work for a company with 15 or more employees and are not a contractor, you may be protected under the American Disabilities Act.

For example, after a colectomy, a person may experience changes in bowel function and require more frequent trips to the restroom. This may be of concern if you work in a role that is highly scheduled, regimented, or requires your availability for long stretches of time. It is important to ensure that restrooms are accessible and available when needed to prevent discomfort and potential accidents.

Be sure to put any workplace accommodation requests in writing; reach out to Human Resources for guidelines or questions. Your employer may request your medical information relative to your request.

The laws enforced by U.S. Equal Employment Opportunity Commission prohibit an employer from using neutral employment policies and practices that have a disproportionately negative effect on an individual with a disability or class of individuals with disabilities, if the policies or practices at issue are not job-related and necessary to the operation of the business. It is also illegal for an employer to discriminate against an employee who has a disability in the payment of wages or employee benefits.

Celebrating Life's Events

It's hard not to have feelings of disappointment when you or your loved one cannot fully participate in family activities or celebrations due to the healing process. It may be small, like not feeling up to tossing a ball in the backyard or attending a parent-teacher conference, or it could be a larger event like missing out on a birthday party, choir concert or big game.

Here are tips for navigating family events and activities during the healing journey:

- Be transparent. Keep family members informed about your condition, recovery and any special needs or accommodations you may require.
- Have a backup plan. This includes a plan for transportation if your bowels and pick-up aren't cooperating. It may also include looking into

livestream ways to watch a performance, joining a video chat while watching opening gifts or watching a recording after.

- Be honest about your feelings. Odds are the patient is just as disappointed they can't participate in activities due to tiredness, digestive concerns, pain or other healing issues.
- If the patient is attending an activity outside the home, arrange ahead of time a quiet space and dedicated bathroom if needed during the visit.
- Look at alternative hosting sites such as a church community room, another family's house or park for a family gathering. Even renting a space is worth the cost compared to the joint stress of preparing for and hosting a gathering while caregiving
- Plan your meals. If your condition requires special dietary considerations, plan your meals in advance to ensure that you have safe and suitable options. Consider bringing your own food or speaking to the host or hostess about your dietary needs.
- Make sure to pack any medications and supplies you need to last for the duration of the event, plus a little extra in case of unexpected delays or changes in plans.
- Stay positive and enjoy yourself. Remember, the goal of holidays and family celebrations is to enjoy time with loved ones and celebrate together. Try to stay positive, focus on the good times, and enjoy yourself!

Overall, with some careful planning and preparation, people who are recovering from colon surgery can participate in and enjoy holidays and family celebrations just like anyone else.

Travel

Traveling when you have digestive concerns can be stressful, but with a little planning, it can be managed.

Plan Your Transportation

You may feel more confident driving instead of flying or taking a tour bus because of the ability to stop when needed. Look at your route to plan for bathrooms along the way.

Stay Hydrated

It's important to stay hydrated when traveling, particularly when flying or in hot climates. It's more the case when you contend with short bowel syndrome or diarrhea. Carry a water bottle and drink plenty of fluids to prevent dehydration, which can exacerbate symptoms of short bowel syndrome.

Pack Medication And Supplies

Make sure to pack any medications, supplies or supplements for the duration of your trip, plus a little extra in case of unexpected delays or changes in plans. An extra change of clothes in case of an emergency is always helpful.

Keep Your Bathroom Routine

Whether you are living with an ostomy or simply managing life with a colon resection, maintaining your bathroom habits and schedule can help. Bringing over-the-counter laxatives or fiber supplements may help if you're experiencing constipation while traveling.

In addition, it may be helpful for individuals who have had a colectomy to carry a "Just Can't Wait" card or similar documentation that explains their medical condition and the need for immediate access to restrooms. This can be particularly helpful when traveling or in situations where restrooms may not be readily available.

Keep Your Diet Consistent

It's so tempting to reach for the local cuisine and comfort foods while you're traveling. But new-to-you or richer foods, as well as additional caffeine or alcohol than you're used to, can cause you gastrointestinal distress. Avoid the high-fat fast-food restaurants and plan to cook or pack your own meals and snacks along the way. Include fiber-rich foods and plenty of water. Look at farmers markets or the local grocery for quick options.

Take Care Of Your Body

Just because you're traveling doesn't excuse you from taking care of your health basics. Keep walking or doing exercise at the hotel gym. Stick to your sleep schedule.

Drink your water. Keep stress down. And enjoy the journey.

Holidays

When your family is going through a life-changing experience such as recovering from colon surgery, it's reasonable to adapt your holiday traditions. Prioritize your and your patient's health. Sleep, eat healthfully and work in light exercise. The rest will take care of itself.

Simplify your holiday celebrations. Decide which activities you will skip this year.

Consider making these adjustments as your situation warrants.

Family Events

Decline to travel this year. Or if you travel, stay at a hotel if desired instead of a family member's home to allow for more quiet space.

Hosting

If you are typically the host for holiday events, consider ordering in a meal, having a potluck or asking guests to stay at a hotel to limit extra stress. Use disposable items instead of the fancy dishes that can't go into the dishwasher.

When you host gatherings, arrange for a quiet space for the patient, and even you, to rest. Be specific in what you need in advance. If guests are at your home for an extended period of time, have a list of possible outings they can go on so you can take a break from playing host.

Minimize holiday meals. Have each family member choose the one dish they can't live without, and keep your meal to that. Spread out dishes among multiple meals, instead of having one great feast.

Create a wish list of things that would help you. This may include respite help or small chores to allow visitors to feel useful.

Traditions

Enjoy your family traditions in moderation. Make one or two batches of cookies instead of eight, for example. Cut back on the amount of holiday decorations or put up a pre-decorated tree. Eliminate holiday cards or send to a reduced mailing list.

Cut back on holiday shopping, and order gifts wrapped and shipped to their destination.

Carve out time for your favorite music, television special or movie.

Have a family game night or cookie decorating party.

Do focus on the time you spent together - instead of the time you needed to be apart. Remind your family members, it was great to see them. Most importantly, embrace gratitude.

CONCLUSION

The initial news of needing a colon resection can be overwhelming. But remember, it truly is a team effort. You have the support of your surgeon, your nursing care team, your primary care doctor, and most importantly, your friends and family. They are here for your questions, your support, and even your tougher days. Don't ever be afraid to speak up.

Recovery from colon resection surgery may not always be as smooth or as simple as you had hoped, but it is manageable, and with a few tools and strategies, your family can get through the surgery process in a much less stressful way.

In Gratitude

To my husband, to whom I promised to live in sickness and in health. I'm so much looking forward to our adventures in health.

To my children, who challenge and encourage me in unexpected ways. I love you. And thank you for not grouching about doing the dishes while I wrote.

To Drs. Maun and Parishak and the surgery and inpatient teams at Franciscan Health. Thank you for caring for my husband and a most unusual case.

To Jan McManus, our Mr. Feeney, who I would take for the high school years if I could. Thank you for teaching my child, for editing the first edition of my book and for being my friend.

To my cheerleaders who encouraged me through this crazy medical journey and the writing of this book. Lani, Jill, Jenny, Christy, Lindsey, Erin, Nina, Aunt Kathi, Paula, Sherri and Natalie. Anyone I've missed, please forgive me. Words can not express the gifts you are to this world.

And lastly, dear reader, to you. Thank you for loving your family enough to want to help them through this medical challenge. God bless.

SOURCES

All sites last reviewed March 2023.

Caregiving

AARP Family Caregiving. (2020, May). Caregiving in the U.S.
https://www.caregiving.org/wp-content/
uploads/2021/01/full-report-caregiving-in-the-united-
states-01-21.pdf

American Medical Association. (n.d.). Caregiver self-assessment questionnaire . https://www.caregiving.org/
wp-content/uploads/2010/11/
caregiverselfassessment_english.pdf

American Psychological Association. (2017, Feb. 9).
Taking Care Of You. https://www.apa.org/pi/about/
publications/caregivers/consumers/taking-care-you

American Psychological Association. (2012, Jan. 11). Stress
in America: Our Health At Risk.
https://www.apa.org/news/press/releases/stress/2011/
final-2011.pdf

CDC and National Association of Chronic Disease Directors.
(2018). Caregiving for Family and Friends: A Public Health
Issue.   https://www.cdc.gov/aging/agingdata/docs/

caregiver-brief-508.pdf

Feinberg, Lynn Friss, Skufca, Laura. (2020, Dec.). Managing a Paid Job and Family Caregiving Is a Growing Reality.AARP Public Policy Institute. https://www.aarp.org/ppi/info-2020/managing-a-paid-job-and-family-caregiving.html

Hasson, Judi. (2022, Jan. 21). Legal Checklist To Help Caregivers. AARP. https://www.aarp.org/caregiving/financial-legal/info-2020/caregivers-legal-checklist.html

Kerr, Nancy. (2021, June 29). Family Caregivers Spend More Than $7,200 a Year on Out-of-Pocket Costs. AARP. https://www.aarp.org/caregiving/financial-legal/info-2021/high-out-of-pocket-costs.html

Schneider, Roberta. (2021). Holiday Stress When You're Caregiving: Caring For You And Your Loved Ones. https://www.amazon.com/Holiday-Stress-When-Youre-Caregiving/dp/B09L4SSZFR/

Singleton, Amanda. (2021, Dec. 28). What to Know at the Beginning of Your Caregiving Journey. AARP. https://www.aarp.org/caregiving/home-care/info-2021/caregiving-lessons.html

U.S. Office on Women's Health. (2023, Jan. 6). Caregiver Stress. https://www.womenshealth.gov/a-z-topics/caregiver-stress

Woodruff, Lee. (2019, Dec. 5). Finding Joy While Caregiving During the Holidays. AARP. https://www.aarp.org/caregiving/life-balance/info-2019/holiday-stress-self-care.html

Colectomy Surgery

American College of Surgeons. (2022). Colectomy. https://www.facs.org/media/oxcpeo0u/colectomy.pdf

American Society of Anesthesiologists. (n.d.) Smoking and Anesthesia. https://www.asahq.org/madeforthismoment/preparing-for-surgery/risks/smoking/

Bowel Cancer UK. (2018, Aug. 18). Types of Surgery. https://www.bowelcanceruk.org.uk/about-bowel-cancer/treatment/surgery/types-of-surgery/

Cancer Council. (2019, April). Understanding Surgery. https://www.cancercouncil.com.au/wp-content/uploads/2020/04/Uc-pub-Surgery-01-64PP-March-2019.pdf

Cleveland Clinic. (2022, April 24). Colectomy (Bowel Resection Surgery). https://my.clevelandclinic.org/health/treatments/4671-colectomy-bowel-resection-surgery

Harvard Health. (2020, Feb. 20). Coming clean: Your anesthesiologist needs to know about marijuana use before surgery. https://www.health.harvard.edu/blog/coming-clean-your-anesthesiologist-needs-to-know-about-marijuana-use-before-surgery-2020011518642

Mayo Clinic. (2022, Nov. 8). Colectomy. https://www.mayoclinic.org/tests-procedures/colectomy/about/pac-20384631

Medline Plus. (2022, Aug. 22). Total colectomy or proctocolectomy - discharge. https://medlineplus.gov/ency/patientinstructions/000153.htm

Society Of American Gastrointestinal And Endoscopic Surgeons (Sages). (2015, March 1). Colon Resection Surgery Patient Information From Sages. https://www.sages.org/publications/patient-information/patient-information-for-laparoscopic-colon-resection-from-sages/

University of Chicago Medicine. (n.d.). Colectomy. https://www.uchicagomedicine.org/conditions-services/colon-rectal-surgery/colectomy

Colostomy

Cleveland Clinic. (2021, Dec. 21). Colostomy & Colostomy Bags. https://my.clevelandclinic.org/health/treatments/22100-colostomy

Colostomy UK. (n.d.). Caring for someone with a stoma. https://www.colostomyuk.org/wp-content/uploads/2020/03/Caring-for-a-person-with-a-stoma.pdf

Colostomy UK. (n.d.). Exercise. https://www.colostomyuk.org/information/exercise/

GI Society (Canadian Society of Intestinal Research). (n.d.). Ostomies. https://badgut.org/information-centre/ostomies/

GI Society (Canadian Society of Intestinal Research). (n.d.). Sex and a Stoma. https://badgut.org/information-centre/ostomies/sex-and-a-stoma/

GI Society (Canadian Society of Intestinal Research). (n.d.). Stoma Complications. https://badgut.org/information-centre/ostomies/stoma-complications/

GI Society (Canadian Society of Intestinal Research). (n.d.). Traveling With An Ostomy. https://badgut.org/information-centre/ostomies/travelling-with-an-ostomy/

National Health Service. (2020, Nov. 16). Living with colostomy. https://www.nhs.uk/conditions/colostomy/living-with/

United Ostomy Associations of America. (n.d.). What is an Ostomy? https://www.ostomy.org/what-is-an-ostomy/

United Ostomy Associations of America. (n.d.). New Ostomy Patient Guide. https://www.ostomy.org/wp-content/uploads/2020/10/UOAA-New-Ostomy-Patient-Guide-2020-10.pdf

Diet After Colectomy

The Association of UK Dietitians. Probiotics Food Fact Sheet. (2018, June). https://www.bda.uk.com/resource/probiotics.html

Bowel Cancer UK. (n.d.). Eating Well. https://www.bowelcanceruk.org.uk/about-bowel-cancer/our-publications/eating-well/

GI Society (Canadian Society of Intestinal Research). (2001, Nov./Dec.). Compromised Bowel and Diet. https://badgut.org/information-centre/health-nutrition/the-compromised-bowel-and-diet/

GI Society (Canadian Society of Intestinal Research). (2002, Nov./Dec.). Diet for Short Bowel Syndrome. https://badgut.org/information-centre/health-nutrition/short-bowel-syndrome-and-diet/

Gilletz, Norene, Erickson, Mandy. (2012). The Colon

Health Cookbook: Easy and Delicious Recipes for

Optimal Colon Health. https://amzn.to/3ium0SB

Hunt, Katie. (2020, June 9). Probiotics don't do much for most people's gut health despite the hype, review finds. CNN. https://www.cnn.com/2020/06/09/health/ probiotics-new-us-guidelines-wellness/index.html

Khanna, S. (2020). Mayo Clinic on Digestive Health:

How to Prevent and Treat Common Stomach and

Gut Problems. https://amzn.to/3iwdSky

Oregon Surgical. (2008, Dec. 10). Soft diet after resection. https://www.oregonsurgical.com/wp-content/uploads/ Colon_Resection_Soft_Diet.pdf

Financial Concerns

Holmes, Tamara E. (2022, July 27). 15 Public Benefits That Can Help Caregivers. AARP. https://www.aarp.org/ caregiving/financial-legal/info-2017/public-benefits.html

How Family Caregivers Can Get The Tax Breaks They Deserve. (2023, Feb. 7). AARP. https://www.aarp.org/ caregiving/financial-legal/info-2017/tax-tips-family- caregivers.html

Waggoner, John. Getting Financial Assistance for Caregiving Is Not Easy — but It's Possible. (2021, Oct. 25).

AARP. https://www.aarp.org/caregiving/financial-legal/info-2019/financial-assistance.html?intcmp=AE-CAR-LEG-EOA1

FMLA

U.S. Department of Labor. (2015, June). The Employee's Guide to the Family Medical Leave Act. https://www.dol.gov/sites/dolgov/files/WHD/legacy/files/employeeguide.pdf

U.S. Department of Labor. (2013, Feb.). The Employee's Guide to Military Family Leave under the Family Medical Leave Act. https://www.dol.gov/sites/dolgov/files/WHD/legacy/files/FMLA_Military_Guide_ENGLISH.pdf

Mental Health

Berry, D.S., Pennebaker, J.W. (1993). Nonverbal and verbal emotional expression and health. Psychother Psychosom. https://pubmed.ncbi.nlm.nih.gov/8441791/

Britteon, P. Cullum, N, Sutton, M. (2017, Feb. 14). Association between psychological health and wound complications after surgery. British Journal of Surgery. https://bjssjournals.onlinelibrary.wiley.com/doi/abs/10.1002/bjs.10474

Chowdhury, Shabnaj. (2019, Feb. 6). Why Some People Get Depressed After Surgery—Even if They've Recovered Just Fine. Health. https://www.health.com/condition/depression/depression-after-surgery

Ghoneim, Mohamed M. , O'Hara, Michael W. (2016, Feb. 2). Depression and postoperative complications: an overview. BMC Surgery. https://www.ncbi.nlm.nih.gov/pmc/articles/PMC4736276/

Newman, Kira. (2019, May 15). How Caregivers Can Cultivate Moments of Positivity. Greater Good Magazine. https://greatergood.berkeley.edu/article/item/how_caregivers_can_cultivate_moments_of_positivity

Seethi, Meera Lee. (2008, Dec. 1). Does Art Heal? Greater Good Magazine. https://greatergood.berkeley.edu/article/item/does_art_heal

Suttie, Jill. (2015, Jan. 20). Five Ways Music Can Make You Healthier. Greater Good Magazine. https://greatergood.berkeley.edu/article/item/five_ways_music_can_make_you_healthier

Suttie, Jill. (2017, March 17). Doing Something Creative Can Boost Your Well-Being.Greater Good Magazine. https://greatergood.berkeley.edu/article/item/doing_something_creative_can_boost_your_well_being

Yip, Deborah. (2018, May 17). How a Compassionate Caregiver Can Help You Heal. Greater Good Magazine. https://greatergood.berkeley.edu/article/item/how_a_compassionate_caregiver_can_help_you_heal

Return To Normal Bowels

Bowel Cancer UK. (n.d.). Regaining Bowel Control https://www.bowelcanceruk.org.uk/about-bowel-cancer/our-publications/regaining-bowel-control/

Keller, Deborah, and Stein, Sharon L. (2013 Sept.) Facilitating Return of Bowel Function after Colorectal Surgery: Alvimopan and Gum Chewing. Clinics in Colon and Rectal Surgery. https://www.ncbi.nlm.nih.gov/pmc/articles/PMC3747279/

Short Bowel Syndrome

GI Society (Canadian Society of Intestinal Research). (2002, Nov./Dec.). Diet for Short Bowel Syndrome. https://badgut.org/information-centre/health-nutrition/short-bowel-syndrome-and-diet/

International Foundation for Gastrointestinal Disorders. (2023, Feb.). Short Bowel Syndrome. https://iffgd.org/gi-disorders/short-bowel-syndrome-2/short-bowel-syndrome/

National Institute of DIabetes and Digestive and Kidney Diseases. (2015, July). Short Bowel Syndrome. https://www.niddk.nih.gov/health-information/digestive-diseases/short-bowel-syndrome

Sleep

Klemann, Nina, Voigt Hansen, Melissa, Gögenur, Ismail. (2015, April). Danish Medical Journal. Factors affecting post-operative sleep in patients undergoing colorectal surgery – a systematic review. https://pubmed.ncbi.nlm.nih.gov/25872556/

Smith, Tracey J., et. al. (2018, Jan. 23). Impact of sleep restriction on local immune response and skin barrier restoration with and without "multinutrient" nutrition intervention. Journal of Applied Psychology. https://journals.physiology.org/doi/full/10.1152/japplphysiol.00547.2017

Surgery Complications And Recovery

Bowel Cancer UK. (2019, May). Long term and late side effects. https://www.bowelcanceruk.org.uk/about-bowel-cancer/living-with-and-beyond-bowel-cancer/long-term-and-late-side-effects/

Cancer Council. (2021, February). The risks and side effects of bowel surgery. https://www.cancercouncil.com.au/bowel-cancer/treatment/surgery/the-risks-and-side-effects-of-bowel-surgery/

Christl, S.U., Scheppach, W. Scandinavian Journal of Gastroenterology. (1997). Metabolic consequences of total colectomy. https://pubmed.ncbi.nlm.nih.gov/9145441/

GI Society (Canadian Society of Intestinal Research). Oxalate Stones. (1997, July/August). https://badgut.org/information-centre/health-nutrition/oxalate-stones/

Giglia, Matthew D., Stein, Sharon L. (2019, May). Overlooked long-term complications of colorectal surgery. Clinics in colon and rectal surgery. https://pubmed.ncbi.nlm.nih.gov/31061651/

Honen Yard, Delicia. (2013, Feb. 12). Postop warning signs set for colorectal patients. Oncology Nurse Advisor. https://www.oncologynurseadvisor.com/home/headlines/web-exclusives/postop-warning-signs-set-for-colorectal-patients/

Kirchhoff, Philipp, Clavien, Pierre-Alain, Hahnloser, Dieter. (2010, March 25).

Complications in colorectal surgery: risk factors

and preventive strategies. Patient Safety in

Surgery. https://pssjournal.biomedcentral.com/

articles/10.1186/1754-9493-4-5

Workplace Accommodations

Employee & Employer Accommodations. (n.d.). Chron's & Colitis Foundation. https://www.crohnscolitisfoundation.org/managing-the-cost-of-ibd/employee-employer-resources

Introduction to the American Disabilities Act. (n.d.). ADA.Gov. https://www.ada.gov/topics/intro-to-ada/#employment

Prohibited Employment Policies/Practices. (n.d.). U.S. Equal Employment Opportunity Commission. https://www.eeoc.gov/prohibited-employment-policiespractices

Travel and Restroom Accommodation Cards (Printable). (n.d.). United Ostomy Associations of America. https://www.ostomy.org/ostomy-travel-and-tsa-communication-card/

We Can't Wait. (n.d.). Chron's & Colitis Foundation. https://www.crohnscolitisfoundation.org/wecantwait

Workplace Resources. (n.d.). United Ostomy Associations of America. https://www.ostomy.org/workplace-resources/

ABOUT THE AUTHOR

Roberta Schneider

Roberta Schneider, MA, is a former journalist for the Kansas City Star who has spent the last two decades writing for medical and healthcare settings. Roberta has served as a medical caregiver for her family members several times, including following her husband's colon resection surgery and journey with short bowel syndrome in 2021. The experiences inspired her to publish two books: the first edition of Living With A Colectomy: A Guide For Families and Holiday Stress When You're Caregiving: Caring For You And Your Loved Ones. Roberta was named an international finalist for the Digital Women's Carer of The Year Award in 2022.

BOOKS BY THIS AUTHOR

Holiday Stress When You're Caregiving: Caring For You And Your Loved Ones

Available in Kindle and paperback.

More than 6 in 10 of us experience increased stress and fatigue during the holidays. And when you're already juggling the challenge of caregiving, that extra stress can beat you down.

Caregiving brings a mix of emotions, on top of the physical stress. Resentment, disappointment, feeling down, grief or loneliness may be among the myriad of feelings stealing your holiday joy.

If you're feeling more humbug than happy this holiday season, you can take steps to regain your holiday joy and reduce the post-holiday blues. Even before the busyness of the holiday season begins, you can learn to control more of your smaller stressors that sap your joy.

And while this holiday season might not look like it did in years past, you can find comfort and joy even while caregiving.

Holiday Stress When You're Caregiving: Caring For You And Your Loved Ones gives insights and strategies to help with:
Stress management while caregiving
Taking care of you
Having a healthy holiday season
Simplifying the holidays
Cultivating gratitude
Managing holiday expectations
Easing money stress from the holidays
Holiday celebrations involving your care recipient
Resetting after the holidays

Living With A Colectomy: A Guide For Families: Preparing For And Actively Living After A Colon Resection

Available for Kindle only. First edition.

For the 600,000 people who have colon surgery each year, surgery can be life-changing, not just for the patient but for your loved ones as well. This means additional financial stress, dietary and lifestyle changes, as well as helping someone through a surgery recovery process. And that doesn't include the impacts on every child and adult living in your household.

This guide to living with a colectomy is designed to help you navigate the changes as a family.